Easy Somatic Exercises for Weight Loss- -

Stress-Less, Effortless Somatic Moves for Sustainable Weight Loss-

By

Brienne Turner

Table of Content

INTRODUCTION

For many years, people believed weight loss was simply about calories in versus calories out. This oversimplified view led to numerous diets, exercise plans, and a booming weight-loss industry. -

However, recent evidence and personal stories have questioned this calorie-focused approach, highlighting its limitations. This book explores the differences between traditional and more substantial weight control methods, emphasizing the revolutionary potential of a physical perspective.-

In the past, losing weight was often framed as battling against too many calories. We've been told to "eat less, move more," carefully monitor our calorie intake, and strive to always have a calorie deficit. Despite its seeming simplicity, this approach has various issues.-

CHAPTER 1

Understanding Somatic Exercises

What is Somatic Exercise?

Somatic exercises are a type of movement therapy that puts emphasis on how you feel inside your body. Unlike traditional exercises that focus on how you look or specific performance measures, somatic exercises encourage paying attention to your body's internal sensations and reactions. The term "somatic" comes from the Greek word "soma," meaning "living body." This approach to exercise recognizes that the mind and body are closely connected. By tuning into the internal movement experience, somatic exercises aim to enhance communication between the mind and body.-

These exercises usually involve slow and gentle movements, prioritizing awareness overexertion. The goal is to move in comfortable and natural ways, rather than pushing your body to its limits.

The Pillars of Somatic Movement

Somatic workouts stand apart from traditional exercises in several key ways:-

1. Inward Focus: Instead of concentrating on how you look or perform externally, somatic exercises prioritize tuning into the internal feelings of movement. This involves paying close attention to sensations, emotions, and subtle changes within your body as you move.-

2. Non-judgmental Awareness: Somatic activities create a space for curiosity and acceptance. You observe your sensations without judgment, allowing you to be present and connected to your body without criticism.-

3. Gentle Exploration: Unlike the often intense nature of regular workouts, somatic exercises encourage gentle and thoughtful movements. This approach lets you listen to your body without pushing or pressuring it.-

4. Holistic Approach: Somatic movement recognizes the interdependence of mind, body, and emotions. It explores how thoughts, feelings, and experiences are interconnected with physical movement.-

5. Embodied Learning: Somatic movement goes beyond physical activities; it's about learning through experience. It helps discover new ways of being in your body, fostering greater self-awareness and understanding your unique movement potential.-

In somatic exercises, there are various techniques to explore, such as:

- **Feldenkrais Technique:** Focuses on gentle, guided movements to examine the nervous system's function, promoting flexibility and awareness.

- **Alexander Approach:** Helps detect and release habitual tension patterns for improved posture and reduced discomfort.

- **Body-Mind Centering:** Investigates emotional and energetic components of the body through movement, facilitating self-expression and emotional release.

- **Rosen Method:** Combines gentle touch and movement to release deep-seated stress and trauma, promoting emotional healing and physical well-being.

- **Laban Movement Analysis:** Studies and interprets movement patterns, providing tools to enhance coordination, expressiveness, and creativity.

The Impact of Somatic Exercises on Weight Management

While regular weight-loss plans often focus on burning calories and tracking numbers, somatic exercises offer a different perspective. They operate subtly, shifting the focus from external outcomes to internal awareness. -

This doesn't mean somatic practices do not impact weight control; their indirect influence can be significant and lasting. Let's explore how these gentle movements can contribute to a healthy connection with our bodies and food, laying the foundation for sustainable weight management.-

1. Shifting the Focus from Quantity to Quality

Unlike traditional workouts that measure success in pounds lost or minutes exercised, somatic exercises prioritize quality over quantity. They encourage us to look inward, paying attention to the sensations and emotions within our bodies as we move. This introspective approach can provide profound insights:-

2. Understanding Hunger and Fullness Cues

By examining our internal signals, we can distinguish between genuine hunger and emotional cravings triggered by stress, boredom, or negative thoughts. This heightened awareness allows us to make intentional decisions about what and how much we eat, leading to better balanced and nutritious choices.-

3. Breaking Free from Food Obsession

Constant calorie counting and food restriction in conventional weight-loss routines can create an unhealthy fixation on food. Somatic practices foster a connection with food based on sustenance and pleasure, replacing preoccupation with mindful enjoyment.-

4. Dissolving Emotional Ties to Food

Many of us turn to food for comfort, trying to ease stress, worry, or loneliness. Somatic exercises provide strategies for effectively managing these emotions, reducing reliance on food as a coping mechanism, and fostering a stronger connection with our emotional well-being.-

5. Cultivating Mindfulness Through Movement

Somatic movement activities are not just physical motions; they open doors to awareness. By slowing down, focusing on breathing, and observing subtle changes in our bodies, we cultivate a sense of presence and mindfulness that extends to all aspects of our lives, including our relationship with food. This thoughtful approach offers various benefits:-

6. Reduced Stress and Anxiety

Chronic stress can disrupt hormones and lead to unhealthy eating habits. Somatic exercises, emphasizing relaxation and mindful awareness, can effectively manage stress levels, creating a calmer environment for making sound choices.-

7. Improved Sleep Quality

Adequate sleep is crucial for regulating hormones and metabolism. Somatic movements can induce relaxation and prepare the body for restful sleep, supporting proper metabolic and hormonal function.-

8. Body Appreciation and Compassion

Negative self-talk and body criticism prevalent in traditional weight-loss programs can foster unhealthy connections with food and exercise. On the other hand, somatic practices promote self-compassion and respect for our unique bodies, creating a supportive environment for lasting transformation.

Key Differences Between Somatic Exercises and Traditional Exercise Programs

Regular and somatic workouts involve movement, but their core beliefs and approaches differ significantly.

	Regular	Somatic
Focus	Traditional workouts often aim for external results like muscle growth or improving sports performance. The focus is on achieving specific goals, pushing limits, and surpassing personal records.	Somatic workouts prioritize internal experiences over external outcomes. The emphasis is on increasing awareness of feelings, emotions, and movement patterns within the body. This introspective approach promotes self-understanding and acceptance rather than seeking external

		validation.
Movement Approach	Traditional programs usually involve structured repetitions of specific exercises targeting particular muscle groups. The focus is on achieving perfect form and pushing to fatigue.	Somatic exercises are gentle and often non-repetitive. They encourage deliberate, thoughtful movements exploring various pathways and possibilities within the body. There's no emphasis on reaching a precise "correct" form; instead, the focus is on establishing patterns of ease and flow.
Intensity and Effort	Conventional programs often include high-intensity workouts with demanding activities and	Somatic activities are gentle and not strenuous. They highlight listening to your body's cues and moving

	significant effort. The goal is to push the body and induce physiological changes like muscle growth or improved cardiovascular endurance.	without force or resistance. The aim is to cultivate comfort and relaxation within the body rather than pushing beyond your limits.
Mind-Body Connection	Traditional programs typically focus on the physical body and muscular activity. While acknowledging the mental benefits of exercise, the mind-body connection is generally not explicitly examined.	Somatic exercises emphasize the interdependence of mind and body. They recognize how thoughts, emotions, and beliefs influence movement patterns.

CHAPTER 2

Getting Started with Somatic Exercises

Setting the Foundation

Here's a simple guide I put together to help you start with somatic exercises:-

Step 1: Set Up a Cozy Space

Find a comfy spot where you can enjoy Somatic Exercises without disruptions. Look for a quiet place, like a corner in your living room or a cozy nook in your bedroom. Privacy and tranquility are key for these exercises.-

Once you've picked the right space, grab a yoga mat or any comfortable surface. Why? Well, a mat adds a bit of cushioning, making your exercises more pleasant. It's like giving your joints some extra support. Plus, using a mat defines your workout area, helping you stay aware of your movements. If you're not into yoga mats, a thick blanket or carpet works, too – the goal is to feel comfy and secure. So, find that peaceful spot, lay down your mat (or blanket), and get ready to start doing your somatic exercise.-

Step 2: Dress Comfortably

Let's talk about what to wear for your somatic exercise – and the keyword here is comfort! Why is comfy clothing a big deal? Well, picture trying to move freely and do gentle exercises in tight, restrictive clothes. Not enjoyable, right? Wearing loose and comfy clothes is like giving yourself the freedom to move without obstacles. It lets your body stretch, twist, and bend naturally. Somatic Exercises are all about getting in tune with your body, and comfy clothes make that easier! -

So, what should you keep in mind when picking your Somatic Exercise outfit?-

First off, go for clothes that make you feel at ease. Choose loose tops and bottoms that don't limit your movements. Fabrics like cotton or breathable materials work great. Also, think about layers – you might warm up during your exercises, so having the option to adjust your clothing is handy.-

Consider going barefoot or wearing socks with a good grip. It amps up your connection to the ground and smoother your movements.-

Step 3: Choose Your Focus

Before kicking off your somatic exercises, pause for a second to decide on a positive focus. This helps sync your mind with your body, making your weight loss journey more effective. Your focus acts like a guiding star, directing your energy toward what matters most. It's like giving your Somatic Exercises a mission – and it can be anything that vibes with you, like chilling out, boosting body awareness, or easing stress. -

Now, what should your focus be? Totally up to you. If weight loss is your aim, you might align your focus. For instance, focus on nurturing a healthier connection with your body or tuning into how your body moves. It's not just about the physical – it's about creating a positive mindset that cheers on your weight loss journey.-

But there's no right or wrong focus. Maybe you want to feel more chill or simply enjoy moving your body. Your focus is all yours to pick, making your Somatic Exercise routine uniquely yours. So, take a moment, shut your eyes, and choose a spot-on focus for you.-

Step 4: Ease into Motion

These light warm-up exercises help your body shift smoothly into your Somatic Exercise routine. They get your blood flowing, wake up your muscles, and prepare your body for the more focused moves. It's like saying to your body, "Hey, get ready – we're about to do something awesome!"-

Now, let's get down to the details – what kind of moves am I discussing? Keep it simple. Start by swirling your shoulders in gentle circles, tilt your neck side to side, and maybe throw in some easy stretches. These moves might seem small, but they do wonders in getting your joints moving and your muscles warmed up. Gentle warm-up exercises lower the risk of injury, amp up the effectiveness of your somatic exercise routine, and even boost your overall experience.-

Step 5: Embrace Simple Moves

Simple exercises give you a sturdy starting point, making your start with somatic exercises positive and doable. They let you tune into your body without feeling overwhelmed, setting the stage for success on your weight loss journey.-

Consider exercises that involve reaching, bending, and contracting different muscle groups. For example, try easy moves like reaching your arms overhead while stretching your legs and then gently contracting and releasing your muscles. It's not about pushing yourself too hard; it's about mindfully connecting with your body.-

Why does this approach work? Because these moves activate your muscles, improve flexibility, and increase blood flow – all crucial elements for weight loss. Plus, they're simple enough for anyone to do, making your Somatic Exercise routine enjoyable and achievable. Pick simple somatic exercises that feel good for you. Start small, listen to your body, and relish the journey. It's not about complexity but building positive, lasting habits.-

Step 6: Navigate with Clarity

Reading up on each exercise prepares you, offering insights into the movements and helping you make the most of your practice. Precision is key here. Every move in somatic exercise has a purpose, and following instructions ensures you benefit most. It's not just about doing the exercise; it's about doing it right. Picture it like learning a dance. Following the steps, you enjoy the rhythm and express yourself beautifully. The same concept applies to somatic exercises. Being precise in your movements helps you reap the desired rewards- increased flexibility, improved muscle function, or heightened body awareness – all crucial elements for successful weight loss.-

No need to rush; it's not a competition. Take your time. Read through the instructions, understand each movement, and pay attention to your body as you go. This way, you reduce the risk of injury and maximize the effectiveness of your practice.-

Step 7: Take It One Step at a Time

Imagine training for a marathon – you wouldn't run the whole distance on day one, right? Well, the same idea applies to somatic exercise. Starting with a doable routine lets your body adapt to the movements.-

Listen to your body – it's your journey. Progress at a pace that feels right for you. Pay attention to how your body reacts to each exercise. If it feels good, that's a signal to slowly add more exercises. If you sense any discomfort, take a step back. It's not about pushing too hard; it's about creating a sustainable and enjoyable practice.-

Your secret weapon? Self-awareness. It guides you on when to challenge yourself and when it's okay to take it easy. Gradual progression is like leveling up in a video game – it keeps things exciting while ensuring you're always in control.-

So, begin with a routine that feels comfortable. As you become familiar with the movements, gradually introduce new exercises. This way, you'll steadily progress on your weight loss journey. It's not a race; it's a journey, and every step matters. Remember, you're in charge of your progress. Enjoy the process, celebrate small victories, and see yourself grow stronger, more flexible, and closer to your weight loss goals with each gradual step. You've got this!-

Step 8: Wind Down and Appreciate

Why finish your practice with a moment of reflection? Think of it as appreciating your journey. Reflection lets you observe changes in your body and feelings after the exercises. It's like checking in with yourself, seeing how your body responds, and celebrating your progress. This mindful approach adds a holistic touch to your weight loss journey through Somatic Exercise. This is where the magic unfolds.-

Take a few moments to notice how your body feels. Are you more relaxed? Did you feel the tension melt away? Maybe you're a bit more energized or centered. Reflecting on these changes deepens your connection with your body and helps you understand the positive impact of your Somatic Exercise practice on your weight loss goals.-

Now, imagine the cool–down as a gentle farewell to your body after a dance – saying, "Thank you, body, for the amazing work!" Do some gentle stretches or relaxation exercises. It helps your body shift from active movements to calm, promoting a sense of well-being. It's a lovely way to wrap up your practice on a positive note. As you finish your Somatic Exercise session, take a moment to reflect, notice the changes, and enjoy a soothing cool-down. It's like putting a bow on a gift – you've just given yourself a mindful, holistic practice for your weight loss journey. Well done, and keep shining on your path to wellness!-

Step 9: Keep Yourself Hydrated

Wondering why it's crucial to drink water after your somatic practice? Picture it as providing your body with the fuel it needs to thrive. When you exercise, your body sweats – like its natural air conditioning system. But to keep everything running smoothly, you must replace those lost fluids by sipping on some water.-

Hydration is like your secret weapon for overall well-being. It helps your body recover after exercise and supports the benefits of your Somatic Exercise routine, especially in weight loss. How? Staying hydrated keeps your metabolism (your body's engine) running smoothly. It aids in digestion nutrient absorption, and helps you feel more energized overall. If you're feeling thirsty, that's your body's way of saying, "Hey, I need some water!" Listen to your body and give it a high-five for the fantastic job it did during your somatic exercises.-

So, after finishing your Somatic Exercise routine and taking a moment to reflect, grab a glass of water. It's a small yet powerful step toward supporting your well-being and enhancing the benefits of your weight loss journey through Somatic Exercise. Stay hydrated, keep shining, and relish the amazing changes within you!-

Step 10: Stay Committed

Imagine planting a seed in a garden – for it to thrive, it needs water and sunlight. Consistency acts like sunlight and water for your efforts, helping them grow and flourish. Creating a regular routine for somatic exercises lays the foundation for long-term success in reaching your weight loss goals.-

Regular practice boosts the effectiveness of somatic exercises. It's not about doing everything at once or pushing yourself too hard. Instead, it's about showing up regularly, even if it's just for a few minutes each day. Consistency is akin to forming a healthy habit – the more you do it, the more natural and enjoyable it becomes.-

Think of it like tending to a seed; if you water it every day, a beautiful flower will eventually bloom. Similarly, with consistent somatic exercises, you'll notice positive changes in your body, from increased flexibility to a more centered mind. Consistency contributes not only to your weight loss journey but also to your overall well-being. It's a commitment to yourself, saying, "I am investing in my health and happiness every day." So, make it a routine. Set a specific time each day for your somatic exercises, whether in the morning, during lunch, or before bedtime. Be patient with yourself, celebrate small victories, and enjoy the journey. Remember, it's not about perfection; it's about progress. Consistency is your ally on this exciting path of transformation. Keep showing up, keep moving, and watch yourself flourish on your weight loss journey through the power of Somatic Exercise.

Debunking Myths and Misconceptions

Myth #1: Somatic Exercises Don't Burn Many Calories.

While traditional workouts focus on intense calorie burning, somatic exercises emphasize internal awareness and gentle movement. However, this doesn't mean there's zero calorie expenditure. Every movement, even small and deliberate ones, burns calories. Somatic practices indirectly affect weight by enhancing posture, boosting flexibility, and reducing stress, all contributing to improved metabolic function and energy expenditure.-

Myth #2: Somatic Exercises Are Only for Relaxation and Won't Get You Fit.

While some somatic approaches encourage gentle movements, other methods, such as Body-Mind Centering or Feldenkrais, may include dynamic and challenging sequences. They might not involve heavy weights or rapid repetitions but engage different muscle groups, enhance coordination, and foster body awareness. This results in a unique form of fitness focused on conscious control and functional movement.-

Myth #3: Somatic Exercises Are Just for Woo-Woo Hippies.

Somatic practices are firmly rooted in neurobiology, anatomy, and movement research. Pioneers like Moshe Feldenkrais and Elsa Gindler crafted their methods by exploring the neurological system and its influence on movement. While certain practices might incorporate imagery or emotional aspects, the essence lies in understanding the body's biomechanics and the connection between the mind and body.-

Myth #4: Somatic Exercises Won't Make You Look Toned or Muscular.

Unlike traditional weight training that targets specific muscle groups for a sculpted look, somatic exercises can also contribute to a toned and well-shaped body. Better posture, increased flexibility, and heightened body awareness may result in a longer, more aesthetically pleasing appearance.-

Myth #5: Somatic Exercises Are a Waste of Time for Weight Loss.

The impact of somatic workouts on weight loss extends beyond mere scale numbers. These exercises address the root causes of unhealthy weight gain:

- **Mindful Eating:** By raising awareness of internal hunger and fullness cues, somatic exercises help break free from emotional eating and foster a more intuitive connection with food.

- **Stress Management:** Chronic stress can disrupt hormones and lead to cravings for unhealthy foods. Somatic practices provide techniques to manage stress and anxiety, creating a calmer environment for healthier choices.

- **Improved Sleep:** Somatic movements can induce relaxation, preparing the body for better sleep. Adequate sleep is crucial for regulating hormones and metabolism.

- **Body Appreciation:** Engaging in somatic activities promotes self-compassion and acceptance, replacing negative body image with appreciation and respect for our unique bodies. This shift in mentality can translate into better dietary choices and successful weight control

Common Challenges and Solutions

Starting your somatic exercise journey for weight loss might pose challenges for beginners. Yet, with practical solutions, motivational advice, and actionable tips, you can overcome these challenges, ensuring a successful and sustainable integration of somatic exercises. Here are common challenges and strategies to address them:-

Lack of Time

For many beginners, fitting somatic exercises into a busy schedule can be tough. But there's a practical solution to blend these exercises into your daily routine seamlessly.-

Break down your somatic exercises into short, manageable sessions. Fit them into breaks at work, while doing household chores, or in other brief moments. Integrate somatic exercises with your activities instead of seeing them as an extra task. Try gentle stretching during a work break, or practice mindful breathing while handling chores.-

Consistency matters more than session duration. Even brief somatic exercises can significantly impact your well-being and weight loss journey. Start with short sessions, gradually extending as you get comfortable. Build a habit that fits your lifestyle. Celebrate each time you make time, whether it's a quick stretch or breathing exercise.-

Find those time pockets in your day for somatic exercises. The simplicity of adding movement and mindfulness to your routine is beautiful. Embrace this approach, and you'll realize even busy days can include moments of self-care. Consistency, not session length, is the key to lasting benefits to your body and mind.-

Feeling Overwhelmed by Complexity

If you're feeling overwhelmed by the complexity of somatic exercises, remember it's not a roadblock. Everyone starts from scratch, and simplicity is your best friend. Begin with easy movements to pave the way for consistent advancement. Instead of tackling many exercises, focus on mastering one before moving on to others. -

This step-by-step method establishes a solid base and enhances your confidence. Once you're at ease with one movement, adding more complexity to your routine becomes smoother. It's about taking it one step at a time and gradually expanding your somatic exercise horizons.-

Difficulty Staying Consistent

If staying consistent with somatic exercises is proving challenging, set dedicated times for them – make it a firm commitment. Use reminders or calendar alerts to help establish a routine. Consistency is key to forming habits. Picture the positive impact on your well-being and weight loss journey when you stick to your somatic practice. Consistency holds significant power in reaching your health and weight loss goals. By scheduling specific times, utilizing reminders, and envisioning positive outcomes, you actively create a routine that supports your overall well-being. No matter how brief, every session is a stride toward your objectives.-

Impatience with Results

If you are getting impatient with results, setting realistic expectations and shifting your focus to the process rather than expecting immediate outcomes is crucial. Consider keeping a journal to monitor gradual enhancements in flexibility, stress reduction, and overall well-being.-

Recognize that genuine, lasting change doesn't happen overnight. Trust the process, and value the journey as you lay the groundwork for enduring results. The consistent, mindful effort over time leads to meaningful transformations. So, be patient with yourself, acknowledge the small victories along the way, and embrace the journey of positive change through somatic exercises.-

Self-Consciousness

If you're self-conscious about practicing somatic exercises, start by doing them in the comfort and privacy of your home. As you become more confident, you can consider joining group classes or taking your exercises outdoors. Remember, everyone starts at their own pace, and it's crucial to concentrate on your personal growth rather than comparing yourself to others.-

Boredom or Monotony

If you find your somatic exercises dull or repetitive, it's time to add some flavor. Explore various types of somatic exercises to keep things interesting and engaging. Joining classes, trying new movements, or even incorporating music into your routine can excite you.-

CHAPTER 3

Warm-Ups Somatic Exercises

Warm-up somatic exercises prepare your body for the incoming movements or exercises you're about to carry out. Start with gentle stretches and easy movements to wake up your muscles. It's like saying hello to each part of your body before the main event. These exercises improve flexibility, increase blood flow, and get your body ready for more active somatic practices. These exercises warm up your muscles, making them feel comfortable and ready to move.

Mindful Breathing

Mindful breathing is a simple somatic exercise that builds awareness and strengthens the connection between your mind and body. By focusing on the steady rhythm of your breath, you can ease tension, reduce stress, and foster a sense of inner calm.

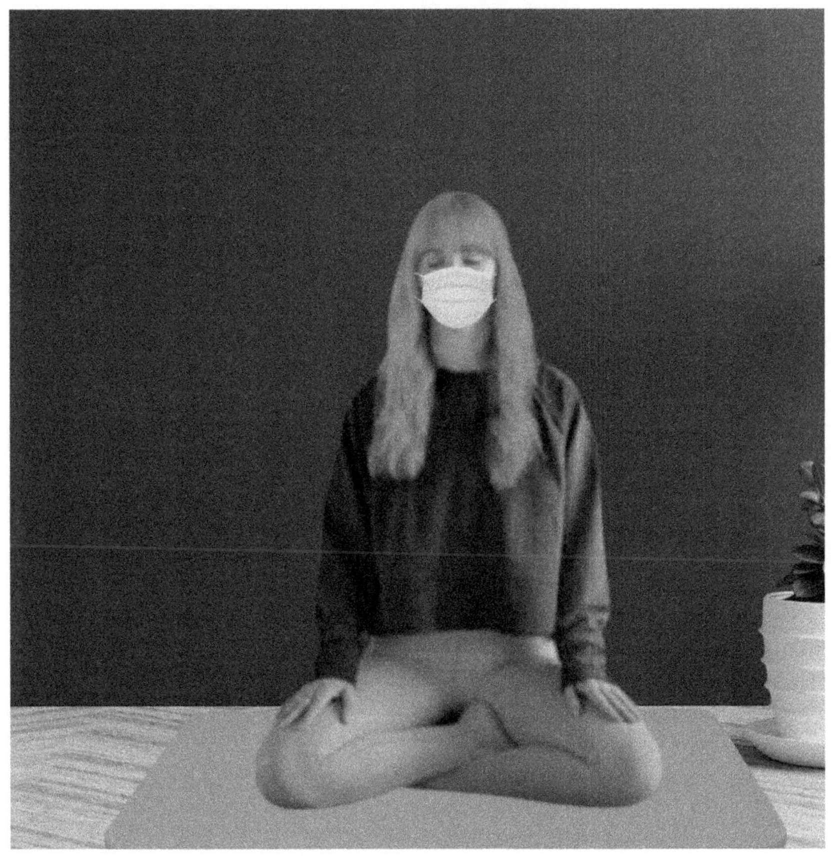

Here are the step-by-step instructions for doing it:

1. Sit or lie in a peaceful place, ensuring minimal disturbances. If sitting, choose a chair with good back support and keep your feet flat on the floor. If lying down, rest on your back with bent legs and relaxed feet.

2. Aim for internal concentration to minimize distractions.

3. Watch the natural rise and fall of your chest and abdomen without trying to control it.

4. Notice the cool air entering your nose, moving down your throat, and filling your lungs. Feel a slight expansion in your abdomen.

5. Observe the warm air gently leaving through your nose, feeling your abdomen softly contract.

6. Allow your breath to be natural and rhythmic. Avoid deep or forceful breaths.

7. Optionally, discreetly count to five on each inhalation and five on each exhale. Helps anchor focus and prevent wandering thoughts.

8. If your mind wanders, gently bring your focus back to your breath without judgment.

9. Practice for 5-10 minutes initially. Gradually extend the duration as you become more comfortable.

Gentle Head Rolls

Gentle head rolls are a straightforward yet impactful somatic exercise designed to alleviate tension and enhance mobility in your neck. When you softly and seamlessly rotate your head, you can elongate and release the muscles around your cervical spine, diminishing stiffness and soreness.

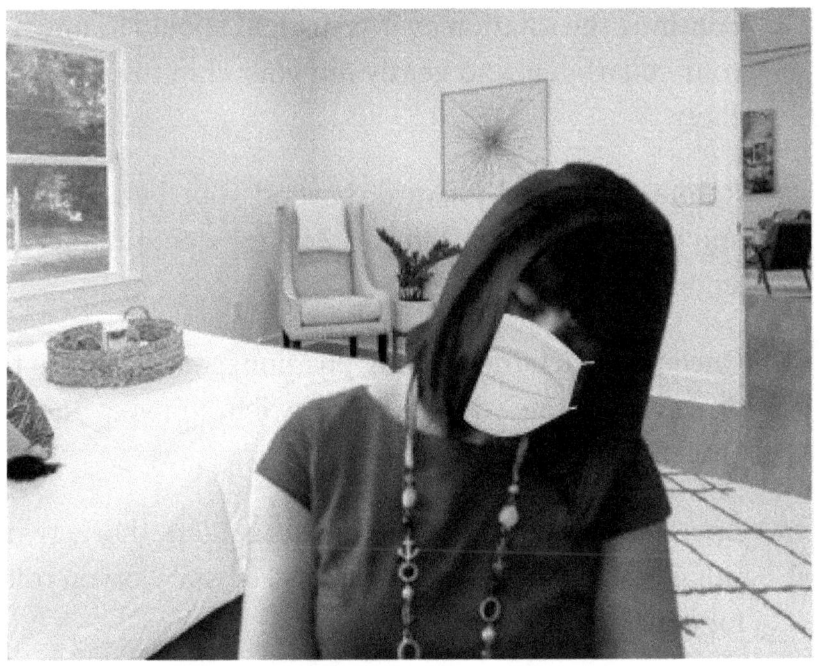

Here are the step-by-step instructions for doing it:

1. Sit on a chair or the floor, ensuring you're comfortable. Maintain an upright posture with relaxed shoulders and a straight spine.

2. Keep your head erect, facing forward. Imagine a gentle pull at the top of your head, lengthening your spine towards the ceiling.

3. Begin turning your head to the right, starting from your chin and moving up towards your ear. Envision drawing a smooth circle with your nose.

4. Continue the rotation over your right shoulder, down to your collarbone, and gently dip your chin towards your chest.

5. Rotate your head forward, beyond your left shoulder, and up towards your left ear. Aim for a continuous and smooth circle.

6. Once you reach the starting position, gently reverse the direction. Rotate your head to the left, drawing another circle.

7. Breathe calmly and steadily throughout the activity. Inhale as you rotate your head back, exhale as you roll it forward.

8. Continue the movement in both directions for several rounds. Feel free to adjust the size and speed of the circles based on comfort.

9. After completing the rotations, incorporate easy neck stretches. Slowly tilt your head to one side, bringing your ear towards your shoulder. Hold for a few breaths and repeat on the opposite side.

Shoulder Circles

Shoulder circles are a basic yet powerful somatic exercise crafted to enhance shoulder mobility, alleviate tension, and fortify your connection with your body. You can stretch and release the muscles surrounding the shoulder joint by gently rotating your shoulders in both directions, promoting pain-free mobility and a comforting sensation.

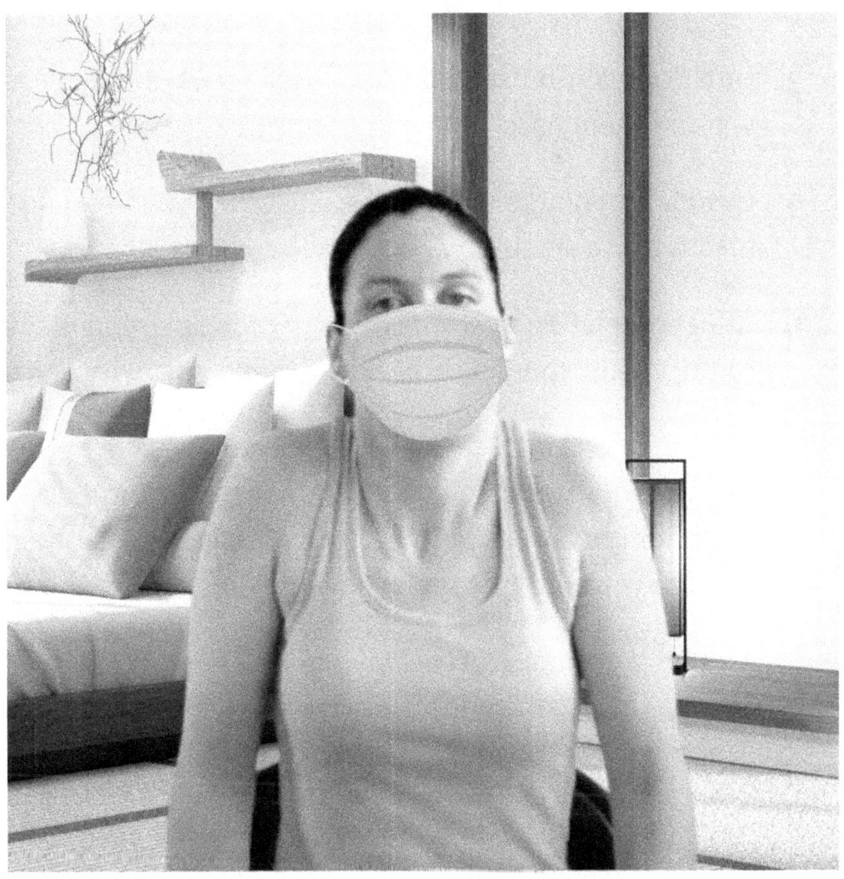

Here are the step-by-step instructions for doing it:

1. Stand with your feet hip-width apart and maintain a straight back. Relax your shoulders, letting them drop away from your ears.

2. Slowly move your shoulders forward, creating small circles with your upper arms. Imagine drawing tiny circles on the wall behind you with your elbows.

3. Inhale as you move your shoulders forward. Exhale as you roll them back.

4. Gradually enlarge the circles, ensuring your shoulder blades move smoothly.

5. After completing forward circles, switch direction. Begin rolling your shoulders backward, starting with small circles.

6. Be mindful of any feelings in your shoulders and upper back. Identify areas of tension or stiffness and let them relax as you continue the movement.

7. Aim for 5-10 circles in each direction. Adjust the number and size based on your comfort.

8. After the circles, include easy shoulder stretches. Roll your shoulders back and down, extending your arms behind your back and holding for a few breaths. Gently stretch your arms upwards and hold for a few moments.

Spinal Twists

Spinal twists are a potent somatic exercise designed to improve spinal flexibility, ease tension, and foster a sense of wholeness in your body. You stretch and release the muscles along your spine by gently rotating your torso in both directions, creating a comforting sensation and supporting better posture.

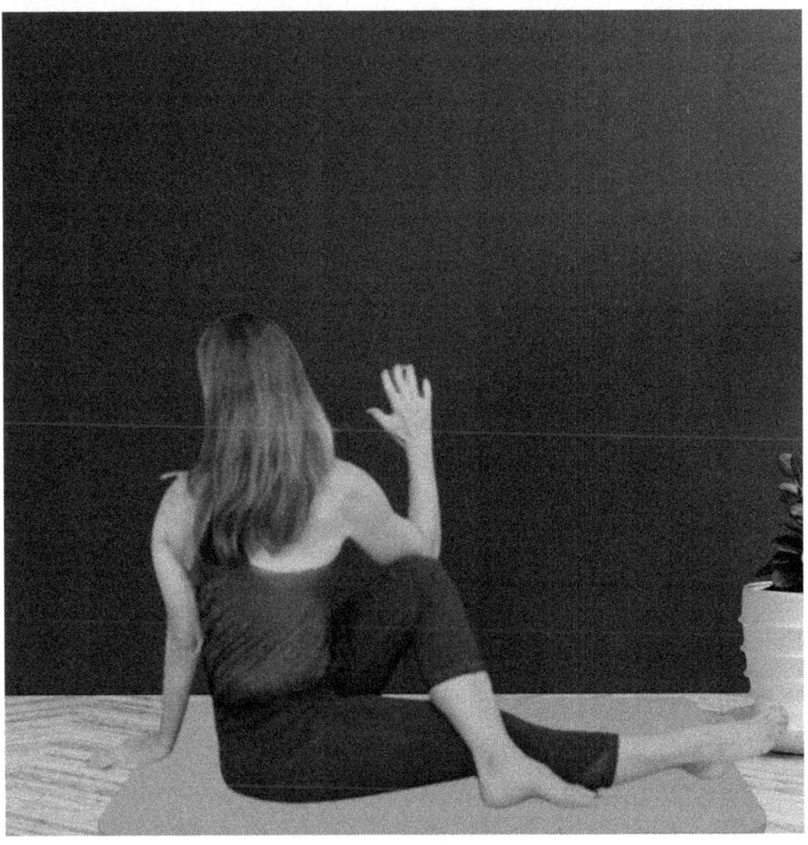

Here are the step-by-step instructions for doing it:

1. Sit on the floor with your legs crossed or on a chair with feet flat on the ground. Maintain a straight spine and keep your shoulders relaxed.

2. Inhale deeply, stretching your spine, and reach the crown of your head toward the ceiling.

3. On the exhale, gently shift your body to the right. Reach your right arm over the back of the chair or place it on the floor behind you. Keep your left arm resting on your left thigh or raised.

4. Turn your head gently to glance over your right shoulder, avoiding straining your neck.

5. Keep calm and steady breathing throughout the twist. Inhale to extend your chest, and exhale to deepen the twist.

6. Hold the twist for 5-10 breaths, allowing your muscles to stretch and relax slowly.

7. Repeat movements 3-6 on the opposite side. Rotate your body to the left and gaze over your left shoulder.

8. After the twists, add gentle spine stretches. Sit tall, slowly circling your back, tucking your chin into your chest, and holding for a few breaths. Arch your back slightly, thrust your chest forward, and hold for a few breaths.-

CHAPTER 4

Somatic Exercises

Wall Push-Ups

Wall push-ups are like a beginner's version of regular push-ups, but they're not just a warm-up. This simple yet effective somatic workout helps you build strength, stay aware, and connect with your body. Using the wall as a friendly supporter, you can discover the power in your upper body, build essential strength, and enjoy moving in a safe and easy way.

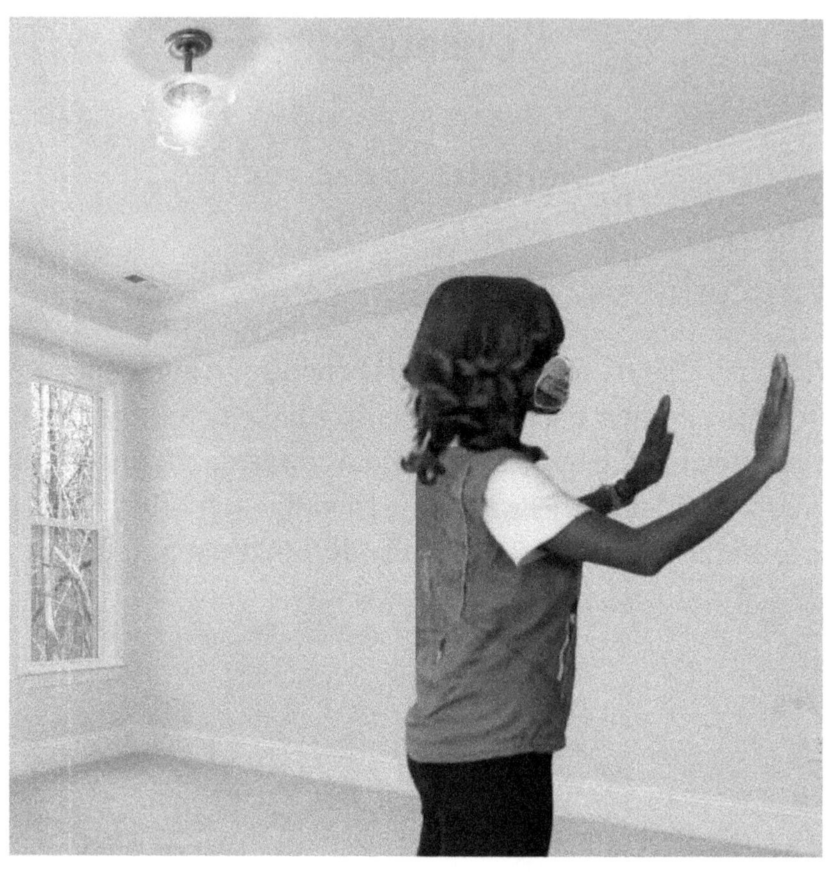

Here are the step-by-step instructions for doing it:

1. Choose a quiet area with enough space to comfortably stretch your arms towards a clean wall. Stand about an arm's length away, leaving room for a smooth movement.

2. Stand tall with feet hip-width apart, feeling rooted to the floor. Engage your core by pulling your navel towards your spine, creating a strong foundation.

3. Take a few deep breaths, feeling your lungs expand and contract. Connect your breath to your body, centering yourself in the present moment.

4. Extend your arms forward, placing hands shoulder-width apart on the wall at chest height. Angle your fingers slightly inwards. Drag your shoulder blades down and back, activating your upper back muscles.

5. Inhale as you gently bend your elbows, lowering your chest toward the wall. Keep your back straight, core engaged, and your eyes fixed just above eye level. Feel the stretch in your chest and engagement in your arms.

6. At the bottom, hold for a moment. Explore sensations in your body, noting any areas of tension or weakness. Breathe into these areas mindfully, letting go of judgment.

7. Exhale as you straighten your elbows, pushing your chest back towards the wall. Maintain core engagement and a sturdy foundation. Feel the strength in your arms and the connection between your body and the wall.

8. Start with 5-10 repetitions, taking pauses as needed. Gradually increase repetitions as you gain strength. Enjoy the sensation of your body growing stronger and more connected.

Knee-to-Chest Stretches

Knee-to-chest stretches, a fundamental part of somatic exercises, offer a simple yet profound sense of relaxation and unity. By gently bringing one knee towards your chest, you ease tension in your lower back, stretch your hamstrings, and create a sense of completeness throughout your body. This straightforward exercise goes beyond typical stretching; it transforms into a mindful exploration of breath, sensation, and inner connection.

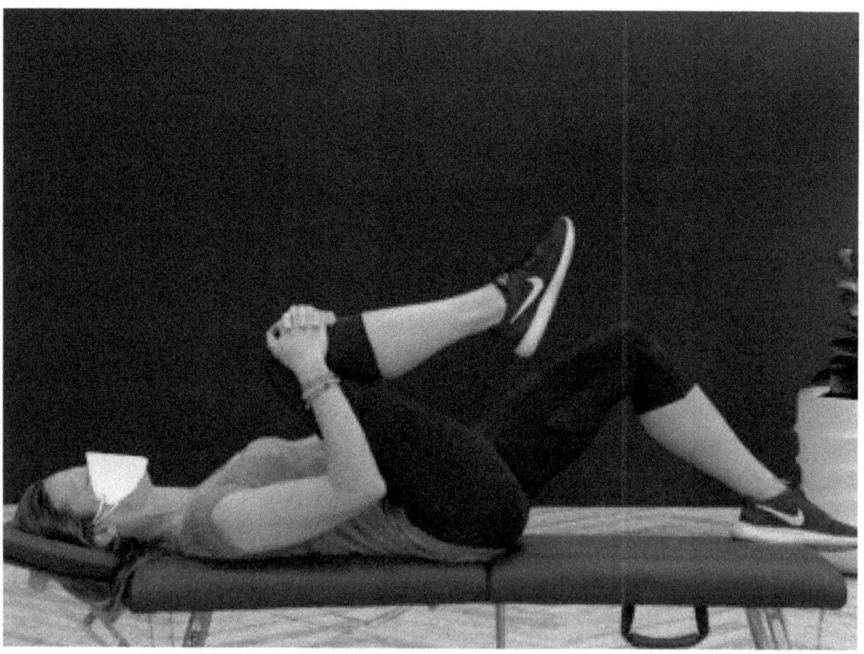

Here are the step-by-step instructions:

1. Lie on your back with bent legs, and feet flat on the floor. Close your eyes or soften your gaze. Take deep breaths, allowing your body to relax into the ground.

2. Inhale deeply, widening your chest. As you exhale, gently bring one knee toward your chest, cradling it with your hands. Feel the natural curve of your lower back against the mat.

3. Notice sensations in your lower back and hamstrings. Accept any tension without judgment. Gradually draw the knee closer, feeling the gentle stretch in your leg.

4. Inhale deeply into areas of tension, exhaling to soften and release. Let your breath connect your spine to your legs, creating a sense of completeness.

5. Hold the stretch for a few calm breaths, allowing your body to yield to the gentle pull. Optionally, gently swing your knee side to side or circle your ankle for added tension relief.

6. Gently release the knee to the mat and take a few breaths. Repeat the process with the other leg, appreciating the unique sensations on each side.

7. After both legs, gently roll onto your side and relax. Feel the connected completeness, the release of lower back tension, and the elongation in your hamstrings.

Arm Circles

Arm circles, often seen as a basic warm-up, transform into a vibrant somatic activity when done mindfully. Gently trace circles with your arms to release shoulder tension, boost circulation, and embark on a joyful exploration of movement. This rhythmic dance forms a symphony of sensations, linking you to your breath and fostering a feeling of completeness within.

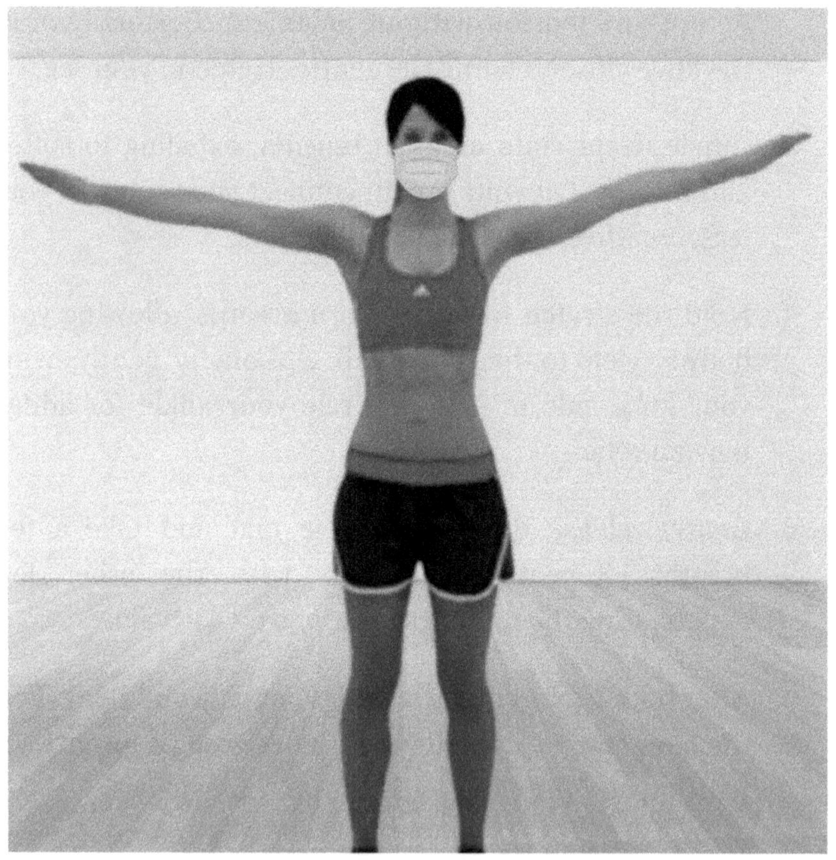

Here are the step-by-step instructions:

1. Stand tall with feet hip-width apart, connecting with the ground. Soften your gaze or close your eyes, taking deep breaths to center yourself in the present.

2. Extend one arm to the side at shoulder height, initiating small, gentle circles. Envision your arm tracing circles on the surface of a calm lake.

3. Notice the sensations in your shoulder, elbow, and wrist. Acknowledge any tightness without judgment. Feel the subtle stretch in your chest and the mobility in your shoulder blade.

4. Breathe deeply in sync with your arm circles. Inhale as your arm rises, expanding your chest. Exhale as your arm descends, releasing tension.

5. Increase the circle size as your body warms up. Explore different directions—clockwise and counter-clockwise— feeling the energy flow through your entire body.

6. Return the first arm to a relaxed position and repeat the dance with the second arm. Observe the unique sensations and movements of each arm.

7. After both arms, stand straight, taking a few deep breaths. Feel the integrated completeness, the release of shoulder tension, and the gentle flow of energy throughout your body.

Jogging on the Spot

Jogging on the spot is a simple exercise that helps elevate your heart rate, promoting cardiovascular health and improved stamina. The rhythmic motion enhances circulation, ensuring better oxygen flow to your muscles.

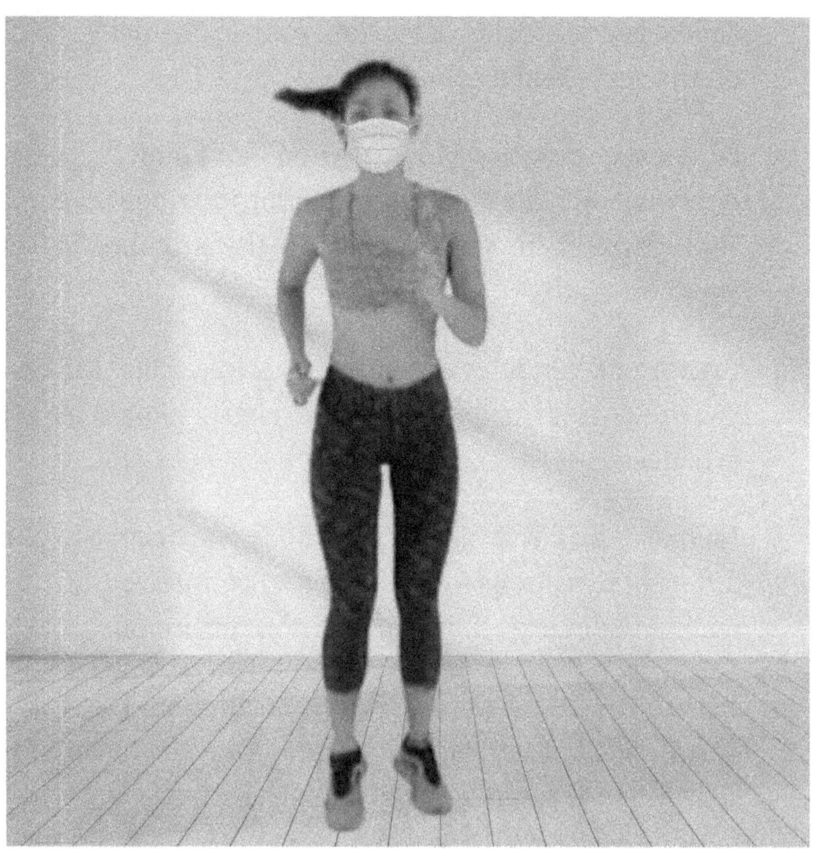

Here are the step-by-step instructions:

1. Stand upright with your feet hip-width apart. Ensure your back is straight, shoulders are relaxed, and gaze is forward.

2. Bend your arms at the elbows. Begin to swing them back and forth in sync with your leg movements. Keep your hands relaxed.

3. Lift your feet off the ground in a light jogging motion. Let your knees lift slightly with each step.

4. Start at a slow pace to warm up your body gently. As you become more comfortable, increase the speed to elevate your heart rate.

5. Maintain steady, rhythmic breaths. Inhale and exhale consistently to ensure a steady oxygen supply during the exercise.

6. Continue jogging on the spot for about 3-5 minutes, adjusting based on your fitness level.

Side Plank Variations

Engaging in side plank variations involves assuming a plank position while rotating the body to one side. By lifting one arm toward the ceiling or modifying foot placement, different variations intensify the exercise. This routine primarily targets the core, shoulders, and hips, promoting strength and stability.

-

The variations challenge balance and engage multiple muscle groups, enhancing overall muscle tone. Aside from the physical benefits, incorporating side plank variations into your routine encourages mindfulness and body awareness, fostering a deeper connection between breath and movement.

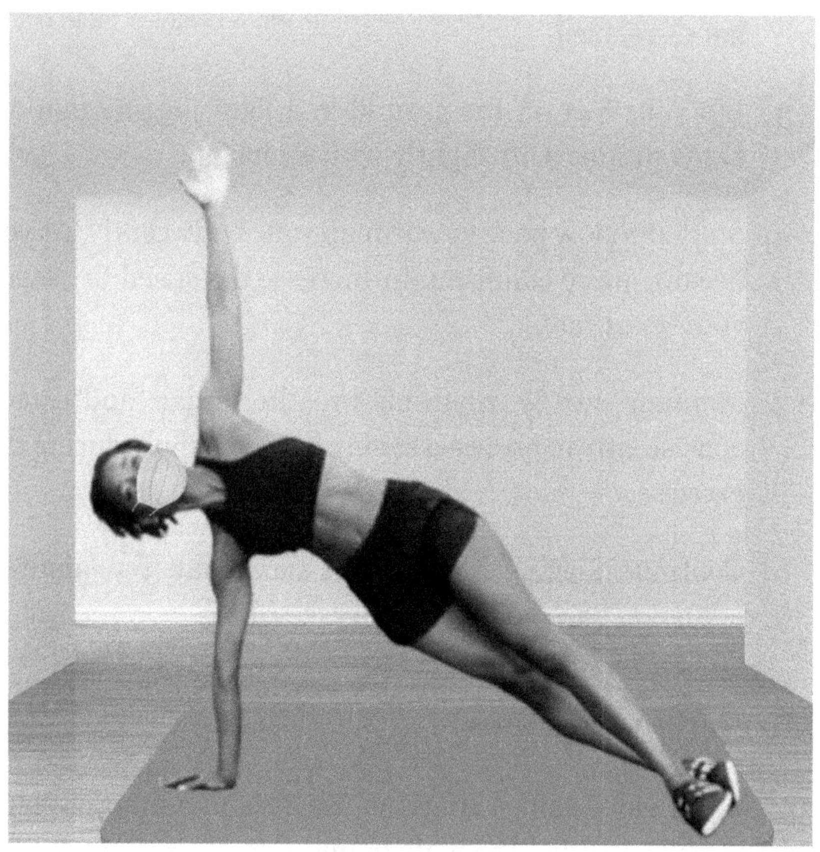

Here are the step-by-step instructions:

1. Begin in a plank position with your wrists directly beneath your shoulders.

2. Rotate your body, shifting your weight onto your right hand to enter a side plank.

3. Extend your left arm toward the ceiling, stacking your feet or modifying with the top foot forward.

4. Hold this position for a few breaths, actively engaging your core and feeling the stretch along your side.

5. Transition back to the plank posture, ensuring a smooth and controlled movement.

6. Repeat the sequence on the opposite side, shifting your weight to your left hand.

7. try different arm postures and leg positions during the side plank variations for an added challenge.

Glute and Hip Flexor Activation

The glute and hip flexor activation involves standing with feet hip-width apart, returning to a lunge, and gently driving the hips forward. This movement targets the glutes and hip flexors, activating these muscle groups. By holding the stretch in the hip flexors and engaging the glutes, the exercise helps improve flexibility and strength in the lower body. This routine benefits individuals seeking to enhance hip mobility, reduce stiffness, and develop a more stable and agile lower body.

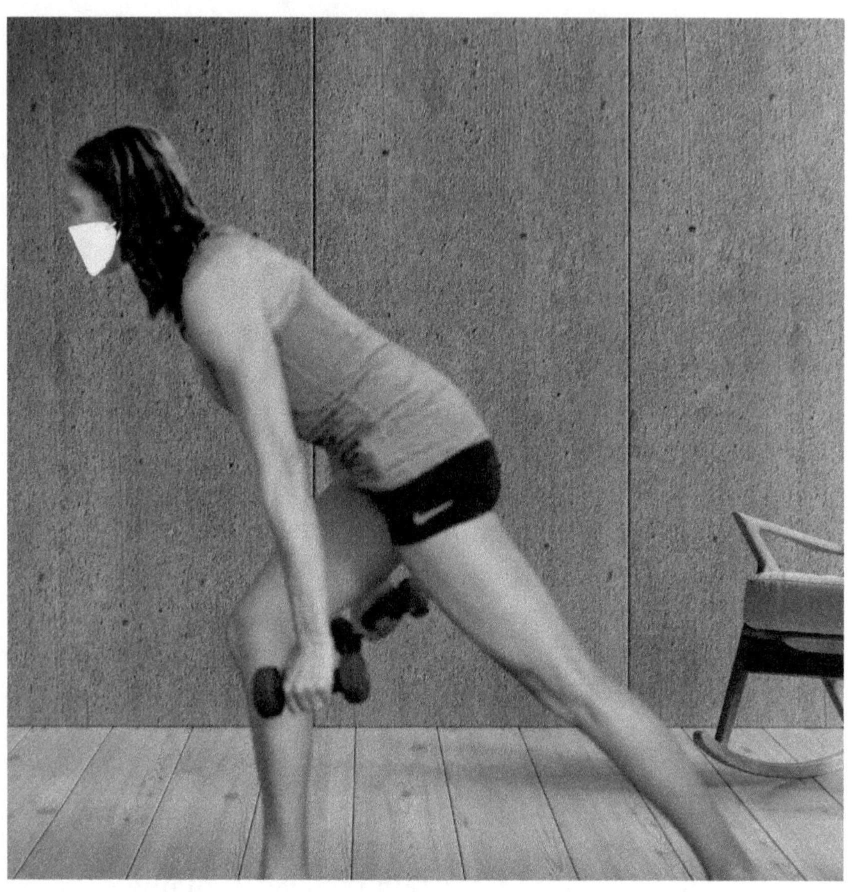

Here are the step-by-step instructions:

1. Stand with your feet hip-width apart, maintaining a comfortable stance.

2. Step back with your right foot, ensuring your left knee is above your left ankle.

3. Inhale deeply, engage your glutes, and gently drive your hips forward.

4. Feel the stretch in your left hip flexor and hold this position for a complete breath cycle.

5. Exhale as you return to the starting position, bringing your right foot back beside the left.

6. Perform the same sequence with your left foot stepping back, engaging your right hip flexor.

7. If comfortable, gradually increase the depth of the lunge for a more intense hip flexor stretch.

Breath Awareness Exercise

The Breath Awareness Exercise centers on paying attention to diaphragmatic breathing, an essential part of reducing stress and promoting relaxation. It encourages a deeper and more effective way of breathing, bringing a calming influence to the nervous system. Regular practice can enhance lung function, lower stress levels, and boost overall well-being. This exercise is foundational in various meditation and yoga practices, highlighting the link between breath and mental clarity.

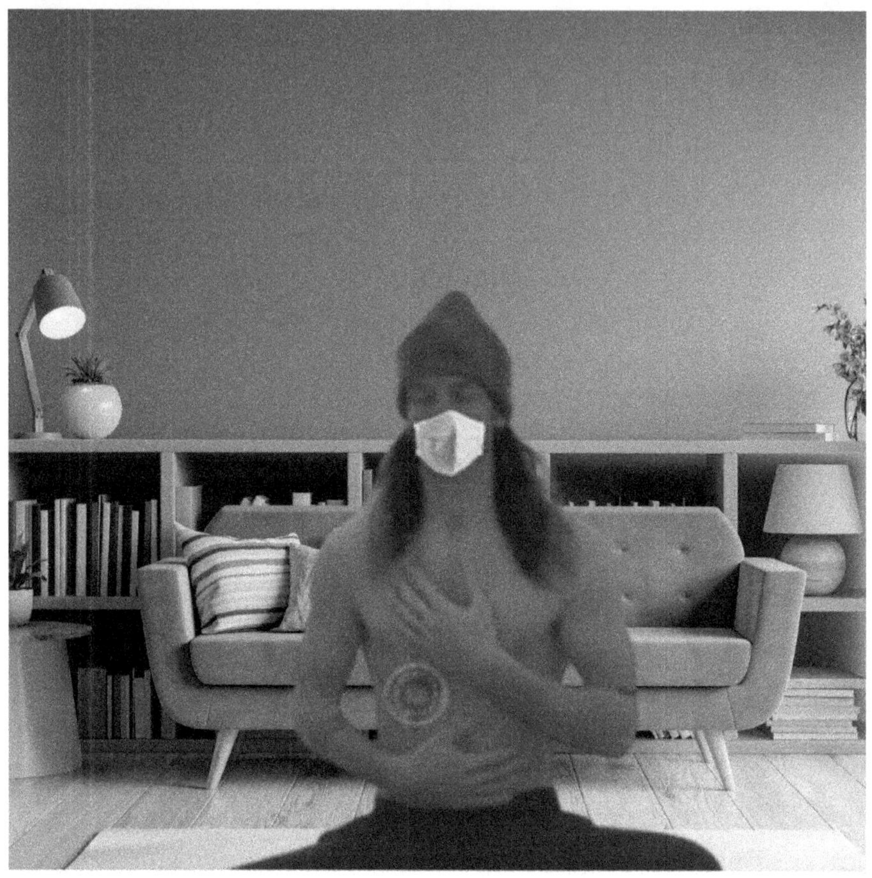

Here are the step-by-step instructions:

1. Start by sitting or lying down comfortably. If sitting, ensure a straight back and flat feet. If lying down, lay flat with legs slightly apart and arms at your sides.

2. Close your eyes to turn your focus inward. Relax your muscles consciously, starting from your toes, moving up through your legs, torso, arms, and head.

3. Place one hand on your chest and the other on your abdomen. This helps concentrate on your diaphragm's movement as you breathe.

4. Inhale deeply through your nose, allowing your abdomen to rise. Feel the hand on your abdomen rise, keeping the hand on your chest still.

5. Exhale slowly and completely through your mouth or nose. Feel the hand on your abdomen fall as you release the air.

6. Continue deep, slow breathing for several minutes. Focus your mind on the breath's sensation, the rise and fall of your abdomen.

Calf Muscle Stretching

Calf muscle stretching involves standing with your hands on a surface for support, stepping back with one foot, and stretching the calf by pressing the heel into the floor. This simple stretch targets the muscles in the calf region. By inhaling and feeling the stretch in the calf and then exhaling to deepen the stretch, the exercise promotes flexibility and relieves tension in the calf muscles.

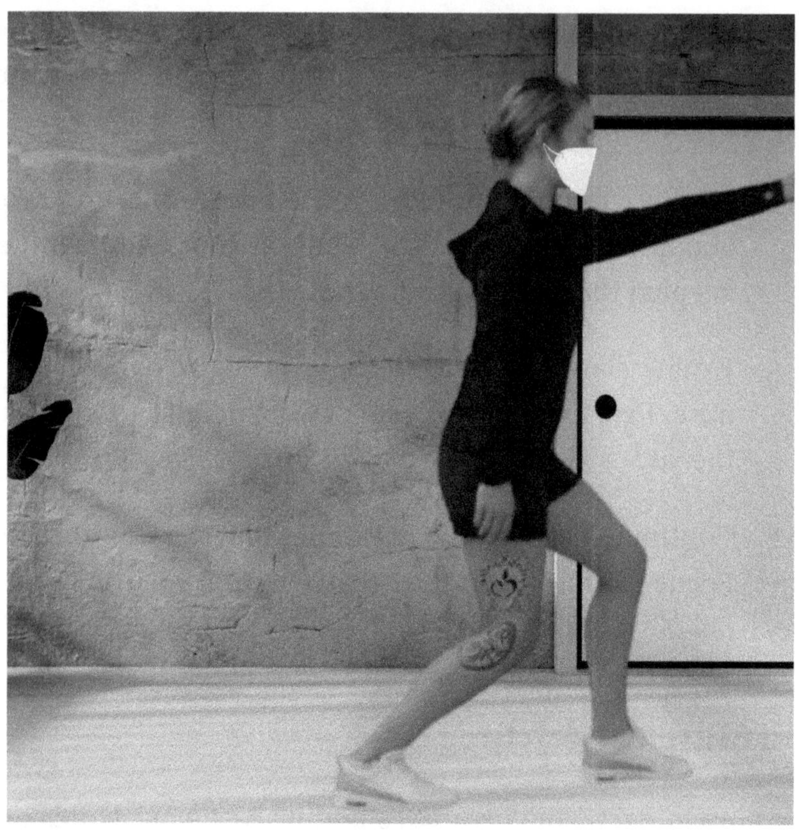

Here are the step-by-step instructions:

1. Stand facing a wall and place your hands on the surface for support.

2. Take one step back with your right foot, ensuring the heel stays on the ground.

3. Inhale deeply, focusing on feeling the stretch in your right calf.

4. As you exhale, gently press your right heel into the floor, intensifying the stretch.

5. Maintain the stretched position for a breath cycle, allowing your muscles to relax.

6. Transition to the left leg by stepping back with your left foot. Repeat the process.

Single-Leg Deadlift with Overhead Reach

The Single-Leg Deadlift with Overhead Reach isn't just about working your legs; it's a graceful blend of balance, coordination, and rooted strength. When you elegantly lift one leg and reach your arm skyward, you're not only toning your hamstrings and core but also fostering a profound connection between your breath, movement, and inner stability.

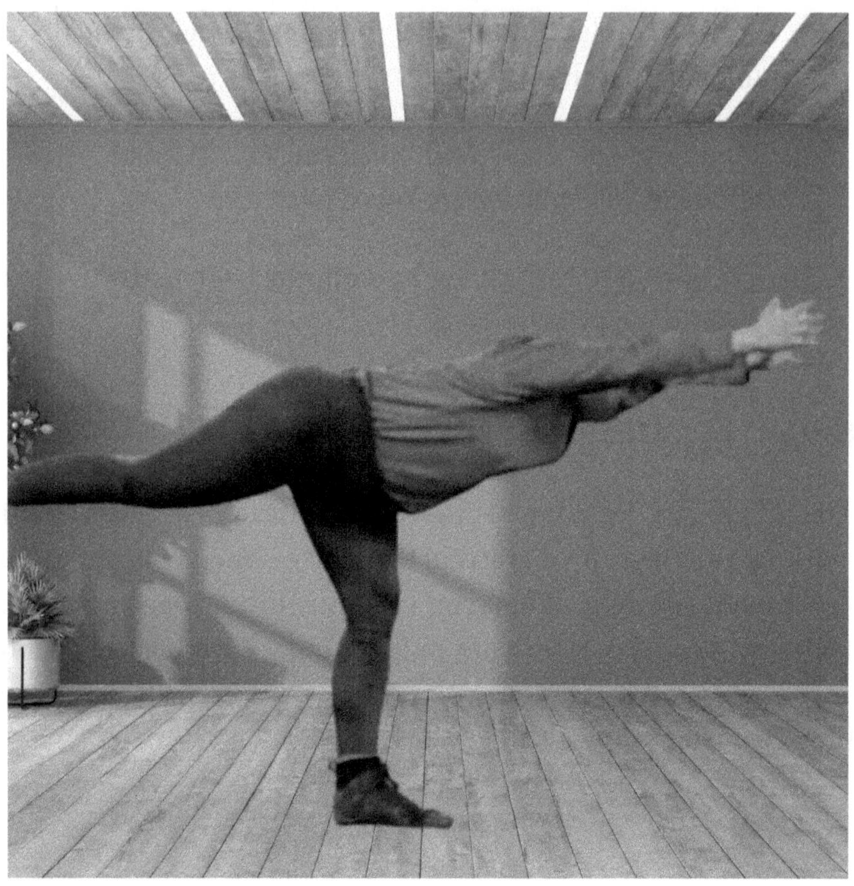

Here are the step-by-step instructions:

1. Stand tall with shoulders relaxed and engage your core. Position your feet hip-width apart, taking a deep breath to center yourself.

2. Raise one leg off the ground, extending it straight behind you without locking the knee. Keep your standing leg sturdy, ensuring your heel remains flat on the floor.

3. Maintain a straight back and engaged core as you lean forward at your hips. Imagine stretching your chest toward the floor, creating a long, aligned spine.

4. Simultaneously, raise the opposite arm straight up towards the ceiling with the palm facing the front. Focus on extending your entire side, emphasizing the stretch through your hamstring, core, and arm.

5. Engage your core and the standing leg to retain balance. Avoid allowing your hips to swing or twist. Maintain deep breathing and control throughout the hinge and reach.

6. Slowly return to the initial posture, keeping your back straight and core engaged. Gently lower the elevated leg back to the ground. Repeat the sequence on the other leg, aiming for 8-12 repetitions per leg.

Ankle Stability Exercises

Ankle stability exercises involve standing with feet hip-width apart, lifting heels off the ground, and returning to the original position. This exercise enhances ankle stability by inhaling during the balanced position and exhaling while returning the heels down. The controlled movements improve proprioception, helping individuals better sense and control their ankle movements. These exercises promote a strong foundation, prevent ankle sprains, and improve overall balance.

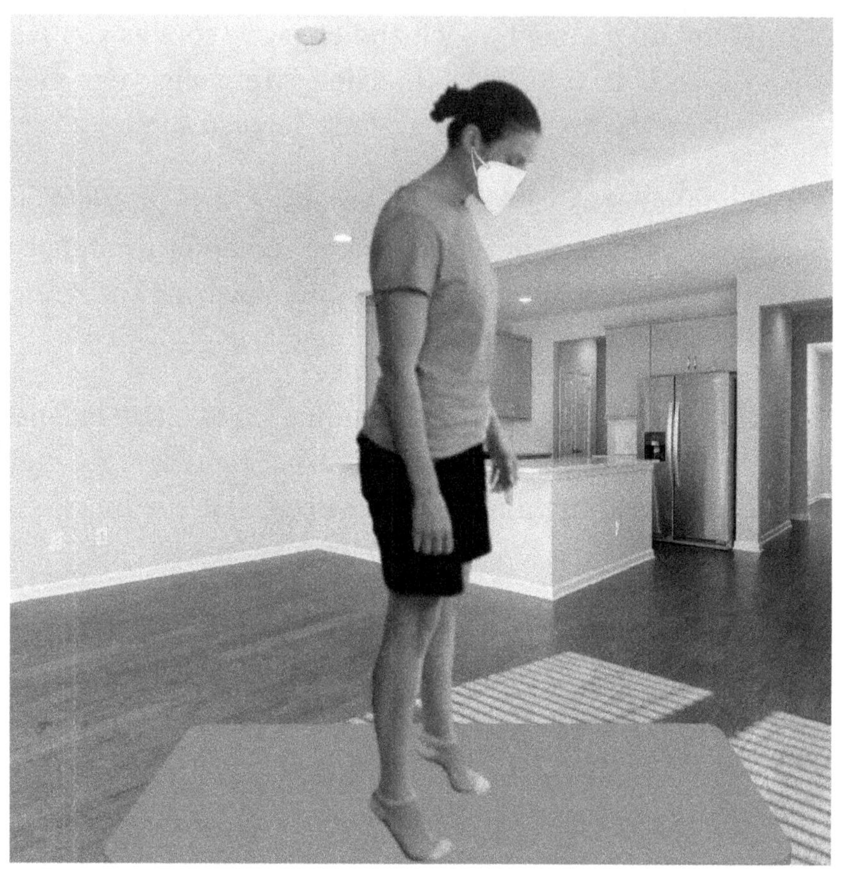

Here are the step-by-step instructions:

1. Stand with your feet hip-width apart, ensuring a comfortable and stable stance.

2. Inhale as you lift your heels off the ground, balancing on the balls of your feet. Engage your core for stability.

3. Breathe slowly as you return your heels to their original position. Focus on maintaining control throughout the movement.

4. Repeat this ankle stability exercise several times, emphasizing controlled and deliberate movements to enhance your stability.

5. To increase the difficulty, perform the exercise with your eyes closed. This challenges your proprioception, enhancing overall ankle stability.

Core Rotations

Core rotations are performed seated with knees bent and feet flat on the floor. These exercises engage the core and work on spinal flexibility by exhaling while twisting the body to each side and holding the stretch. The benefits include improved abdominal strength, increased flexibility in the spine, and a sense of completeness in the body.

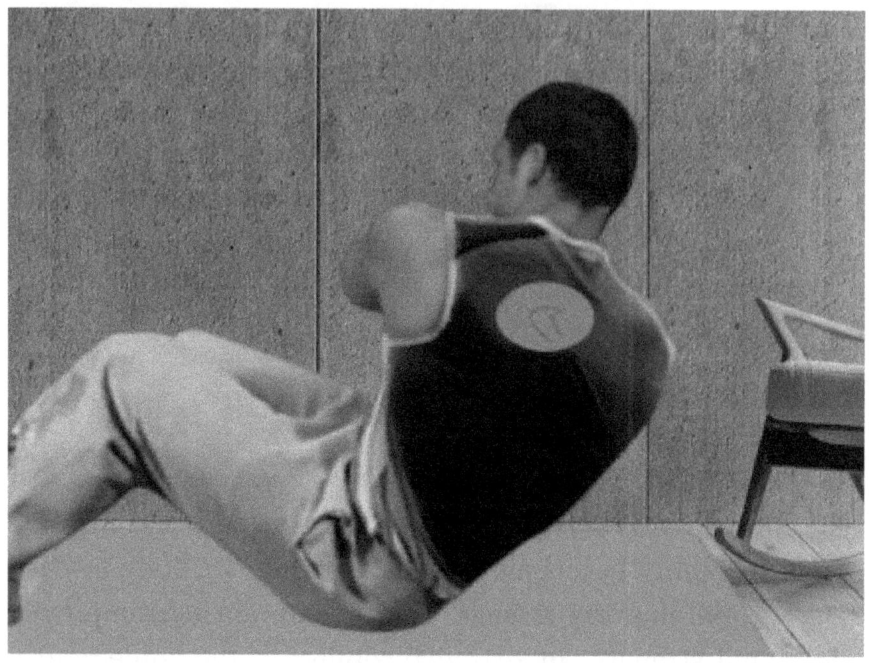

Here are the step-by-step instructions:

1. Sit with your knees bent and feet flat on the floor, ensuring a comfortable posture.

2. Breathe out, elongating your spine to create a tall, engaged posture.

3. Exhale again, twisting your body to the right. Place your left hand on the outside of your right knee.

4. Maintain this position for a breath cycle, focusing on the twist at your core.

5. Exhale and smoothly return to the center, releasing the twist.

6. Now, repeat the process on the opposite side. Rotate left, placing your right hand on the outside of your left knee.

7. Continue alternating the twists from right to left, synchronizing your breath with each movement.

Pilates-Inspired Ab Workouts

Somatic Pilates-inspired ab workouts involve lying on your back, engaging your core, and performing controlled movements to strengthen abdominal muscles. Inhaling to engage the core and exhaling while lifting your head, neck, and shoulders off the mat are key components. These exercises go beyond traditional ab workouts, offering benefits such as improved core strength, enhanced posture, and increased body awareness.

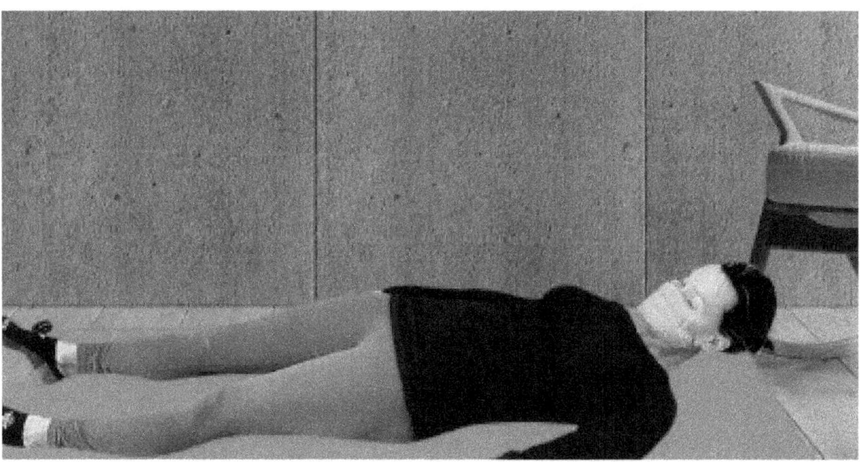

Here are the step-by-step instructions:

1. Lie on your back with your legs stretched out comfortably.

2. Take a deep breath, focusing on engaging your core muscles.

3. As you exhale, lift your head, neck, and shoulders off the mat. Feel the contraction in your abdominal muscles.

4. Pause for a breath cycle, maintaining the lifted position. Continue to engage your core.

5. Inhale as you lower back down and exhale slowly. Focus on controlled movements.

6. Repeat the exercise, adding variations like leg lifts or bicycle movements. These variations add intensity and target different parts of your abdominal muscles.

Squats

Squats are a powerful strength-building exercise focused on muscles in your lower body—quads, hamstrings, glutes, and calves. This move strengthens your legs, contributes to better mental well-being, and tones your overall lower body muscles.

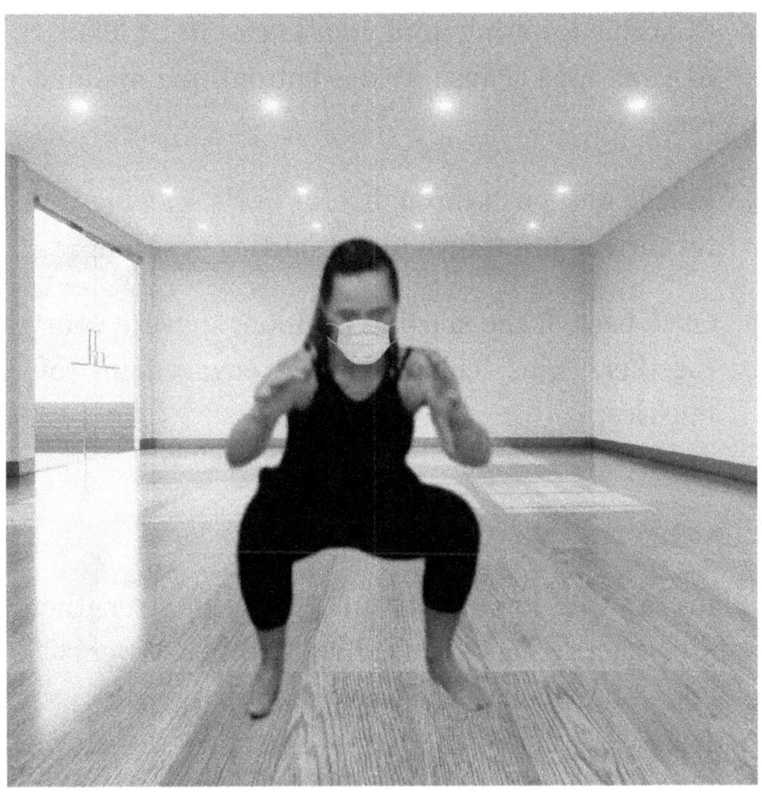

Here are the step-by-step instructions:

1. Stand with your feet shoulder-width apart, toes pointing slightly outward. Place your hands on the back of your head or together in front of your chest.

2. Keep your shoulders back, engage your abs, and maintain a neutral spine.

3. Inhale and shift your weight onto your heels. Hinge at your hips and bend your knees as if sitting in an imaginary chair.

4. Continue lowering until your knees are at least parallel to your hips. Pause at the bottom, maintaining good form.

5. Exhale and push through your heels, moving your hips forward as you return to the starting position.

6. Once back at the starting position, squeeze your glutes together. This enhances the engagement of your muscles.

Plank

The plank is a well-known workout that helps strengthen your core muscles, engaging various groups like abs, lower back, and shoulders. Doing planks is a powerful way to enhance your core strength and stability and boost your mental well-being.

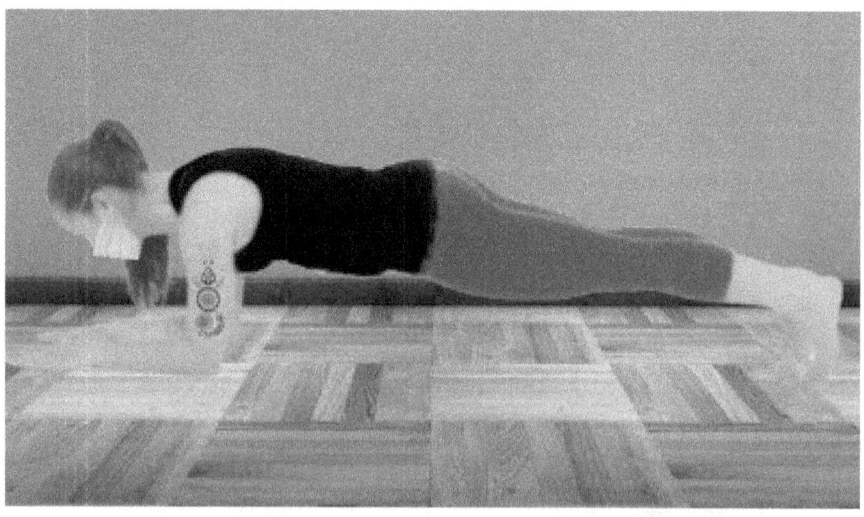

Here are the step-by-step instructions:

1. Get down on the ground. Position your elbows directly beneath your shoulders and extend your legs, supporting your weight on your elbows and toes.

2. Squeeze your glutes and tighten your core, imagining your belly button pulling towards your spine. This creates tension throughout your entire body.

3. Contract your lower back, lats, and rhomboids. Ensure your back forms a straight line—no dipping pelvis or rising butt.

4. Face your gaze downward, keeping your neck neutral to protect it.

5. Maintain this strong position for 10 seconds. Slowly release to the floor.

6. As you get comfortable, gradually extend the duration. Work your way up to 30, 45, or even 60 seconds over time. This exercise is a powerhouse for building strength and stability.

Bridge Pose

The Bridge Pose, also known as Setu Bandhasana, is useful for building strength in your back, glutes, and hamstrings. It also opens up your chest and shoulders, which is great if you sit long. This pose can help improve your posture and ease lower back pain. Doing the Bridge Pose regularly can strengthen your core and contribute to a more stable and balanced lower body.

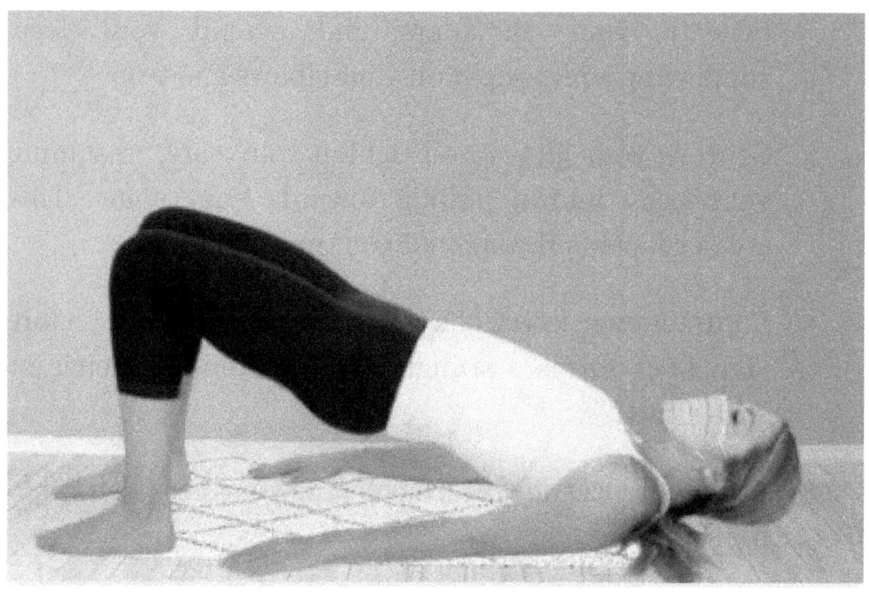

Here are the step-by-step instructions:

1. Lie on your back with knees bent, feet flat on the ground, arms extended alongside your body, palms down, fingertips lightly touching your heels.

2. Press firmly through your feet and arms, raising your hips toward the ceiling. Keep thighs and feet parallel, avoiding outward knee movement.

3. Activate your glutes and hamstrings while lifting, ensuring a straight line from shoulders to knees. Avoid overarch in the lower back.

4. Keep your neck relaxed, gaze upward, and avoid turning your head side-to-side.

5. Maintain the Bridge Pose for 30 seconds to 1 minute. Breathe deeply, sustaining a steady lift through your hips.

6. To exit, slowly lower your hips to the ground. Afterward, hug your knees to your chest for a gentle counter-stretch.

Jumping Jacks

Jumping jacks are a fantastic way to boost your physical and mental well-being. The mix of heart-healthy exercise and rhythmic motion can trigger the release of feel-good endorphins, alleviate stress, and lift your spirits.

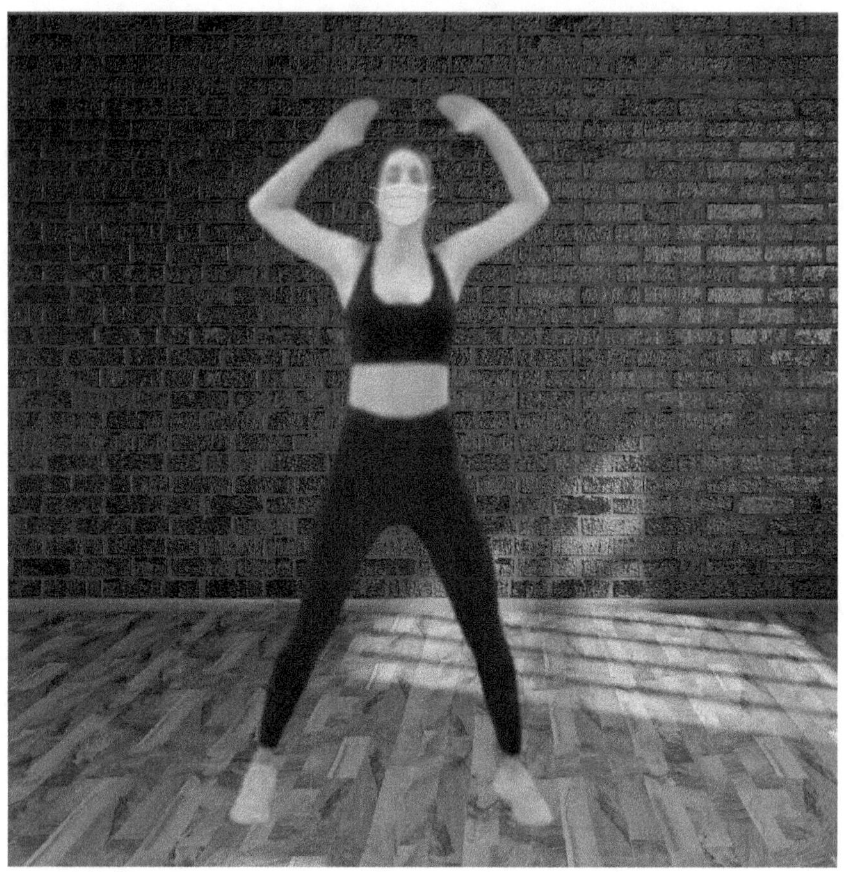

Here are the step-by-step instructions:

1. Stand up with your legs slightly apart, keep your knees relaxed, and let your hands rest on your thighs.

2. Keep those knees a little bent. Now, open your arms and legs to the sides like you spread your wings. At the same time, swing your arms above your head, and your legs go wider than your shoulders.

3. Close your arms and legs back to where you began. It's like a gentle clap above your head with your feet coming back together.

4. You can do as many rounds as you like, but aiming for at least 20 jumping jacks in each set is a good start. It's a simple, effective way to get your body moving and your heart smiling.

Balancing Table Pose

Pilates-inspired ab workouts involve lying on your back, engaging your core, and performing controlled movements to strengthen abdominal muscles. Inhaling to engage the core and exhaling while lifting your head, neck, and shoulders off the mat are key components. These exercises go beyond traditional ab workouts, offering benefits such as improved core strength, enhanced posture, and increased body awareness. Incorporating variations like leg lifts or bicycle movements provides a well-rounded workout for the entire abdominal region.

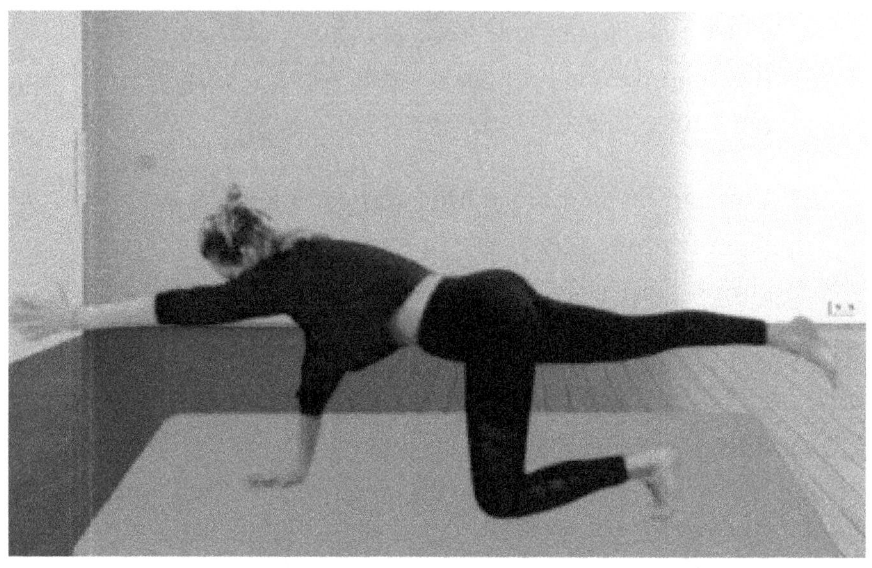

-

Here are the step-by-step instructions:

1. Begin on your hands and knees in a tabletop position, ensuring your wrists are under your shoulders and knees under your hips. Keep your back flat and look down at the floor.

2. Reach your right arm forward in line with your torso while simultaneously extending your left leg back, maintaining parallel alignment to the floor.

3. Engage your core muscles to stay balanced. Keep your hips and shoulders squared to the floor.

4. Maintain the position for a few seconds, emphasizing stability and balance.

5. Gently lower your extended arm and leg back to the tabletop position.

6. Extend your left arm and right leg, following the same steps. Alternate sides for several repetitions.

Lunge with a Twist

The Lunge with a Twist is a workout that blends stretching and movement. It focuses on your legs, hips, and spine muscles, giving you a dynamic stretch to boost flexibility and promote torso mobility. This exercise is especially good for easing tension in tight hip flexors and enhancing the rotational movement of your upper body. It's an excellent choice for including in your warm-up or cool-down routine.

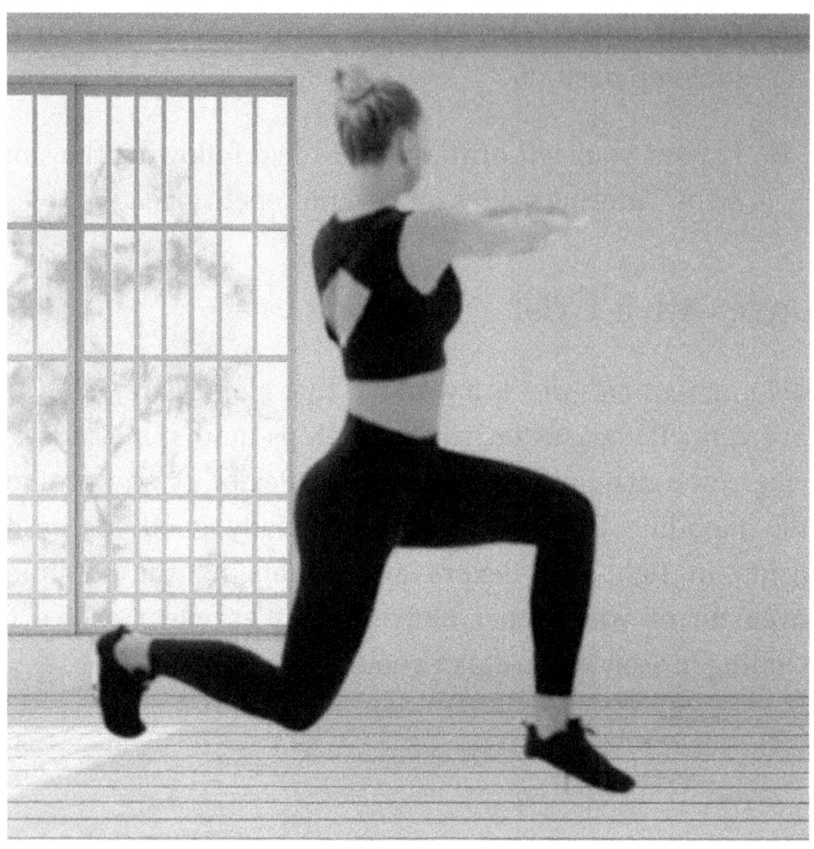

Here are the step-by-step instructions:

1. Stand with feet together, hands on hips, shoulders relaxed, and back straight.

2. Take a sizable step forward with your right foot, bending the knee to approximately 90 degrees. Ensure the front thigh is parallel to the floor and the back leg is straight with the heel lifted.

3. Extend your arms to the sides at shoulder height while lunging. Twist your upper body to the right, keeping your arms parallel to the floor. Optionally, turn your head to look over your right shoulder.

4. Untwist your upper body, bringing arms back to your sides. Push off your right foot to return to the starting position.

5. Step forward with your left foot, twisting to the left this time.

6. Coordinate your movements with your breath. Inhale as you step into the lunge and exhale as you twist. Repeat for desired repetitions.-

CHAPTER 5

28-Day Workout Plan

Week 1

Day 1

Warm Up Exercise: Mindful Breathing

Somatic Exercises	Reps
Wall Push-Ups	15 reps
Knee-to-Chest Stretches (both sides)	12 reps each side
Arm Circles	20 reps
Jogging on the Spot	3 minutes
Side Plank Variations (both sides)	30 seconds each side

Day 2

Warm Up Exercise: Gentle Head Rolls

Somatic Exercises	Reps
Glute and Hip Flexor Activation	15 reps each leg
Breath Awareness Exercise	5 minutes
Calf Muscle Stretching (both sides)	15 seconds each side
Single-Leg Deadlift with Overhead Reach (both sides)	12 reps each side
Ankle Stability Exercises	15 reps
Core Rotations (both sides)	15 reps each side

Day 3

Warm Up Exercise: Shoulder Circles

Somatic Exercises	Reps

Pilates-Inspired Ab Workouts	15 reps
Squats	20 reps
Lunge with a Twist (both sides)	12 reps each side
Plank	30 seconds
Bridge Pose	20 seconds
Jumping Jacks	3 minutes

Day 4

Warm Up Exercise: Spinal Twists

Somatic Exercises	Reps
Balancing Table Pose (both sides)	15 reps each side
Lunge with a Twist (both	12 reps each side

sides)	
Wall Push-Ups	15 reps
Knee-to-Chest Stretches (both sides)	12 reps each side
Arm Circles	20 reps
Jogging on the Spot	3 minutes

Day 5

Warm Up Exercise: Mindful Breathing

Somatic Exercises	Reps
Side Plank Variations (both sides)	30 seconds each side
Glute and Hip Flexor Activation	15 reps each leg
Breath Awareness Exercise	5 minutes

Calf Muscle Stretching (both sides)	15 seconds each side
Single-Leg Deadlift with Overhead Reach (both sides)	12 reps each side

Day 6

Warm Up Exercise: Gentle Head Rolls

Somatic Exercises	Reps
Ankle Stability Exercises	15 reps
Core Rotations (both sides)	15 reps each side
Pilates-Inspired Ab Workouts	15 reps
Squats	20 reps
Lunge with a Twist (both sides)	12 reps each side

Plank	30 seconds

Day 7

Warm Up Exercise: Shoulder Circles

Somatic Exercises	Reps
Bridge Pose	20 seconds
Jumping Jacks	3 minutes
Balancing Table Pose (both sides)	15 reps each side
Lunge with a Twist (both sides)	12 reps each side
Wall Push-Ups	15 reps
Knee-to-Chest Stretches (both sides)	12 reps each side

Week 2

Day 8

Warm Up Exercise: Spinal Twists

Somatic Exercises	Reps
Arm Circles	20 reps
Jogging on the Spot	3 minutes
Side Plank Variations (both sides)	30 seconds each side
Glute and Hip Flexor Activation	15 reps each leg
Breath Awareness Exercise	5 minutes

Day 9

Warm Up Exercise: Mindful Breathing

Somatic Exercises	Reps

Calf Muscle Stretching (both sides)	15 reps each side
Single-Leg Deadlift with Overhead Reach (both sides)	12 reps each side
Ankle Stability Exercises	15 reps
Core Rotations (both sides)	15 reps each side
Pilates-Inspired Ab Workouts	15 reps
Squats	20 reps

Day 10

Warm Up Exercise: Gentle Head Rolls

Somatic Exercises	Reps
Plank	30 seconds
Bridge Pose	20 seconds

Jumping Jacks	3 minutes
Balancing Table Pose (both sides)	15 reps each side
Lunge with a Twist (both sides)	12 reps each side

Day 11

Warm Up Exercise: Shoulder Circles

Somatic Exercises	Reps
Wall Push-Ups	20 reps
Knee-to-Chest Stretches (both sides)	15 reps each side
Arm Circles	20 reps
Jogging on the Spot	3 minutes
Side Plank Variations (both	30 seconds each side

sides)	

Day 12

Warm Up Exercise: Spinal Twists

Somatic Exercises	Reps
Glute and Hip Flexor Activation (both sides)	15 reps each side
Breath Awareness Exercise	5 minutes
Calf Muscle Stretching (both sides)	15 seconds each side
Single-Leg Deadlift with Overhead Reach (both sides)	12 reps each side
Ankle Stability Exercises	15 reps
Core Rotations (both sides)	15 reps each side

Day 13

Warm Up Exercise: Mindful Breathing

Somatic Exercises	Reps
Pilates-Inspired Ab Workouts	15 reps
Squats	20 reps
Lunge with a Twist (both sides)	12 reps each side
Plank	30 seconds
Bridge Pose	20 seconds
Jumping Jacks	3 minutes

Day 14

Warm Up Exercise: Gentle Head Rolls

Somatic Exercises	Reps

Balancing Table Pose (both sides)	12 reps each side
Lunge with a Twist (both sides)	10 reps each side
Mindful Breathing	5 minutes
Wall Push-Ups	25 reps
Knee-to-Chest Stretches (both sides)	18 reps each side
Arm Circles	25 reps

Week 3

Day 15

Warm Up Exercise: Shoulder Circles

Somatic Exercises	Reps
Jogging on the Spot	5 minutes

Side Plank Variations (both sides)	25 seconds each side
Glute and Hip Flexor Activation (both sides)	18 reps each side
Breath Awareness Exercise	6 minutes
Calf Muscle Stretching (both sides)	20 seconds each side

Day 16

Warm Up Exercise: Spinal Twists

Somatic Exercises	Reps
Single-Leg Deadlift with Overhead Reach (both sides)	15 reps each side
Ankle Stability Exercises	18 reps
Core Rotations (both sides)	18 reps each side

Pilates-Inspired Ab Workouts	18 reps
Squats	25 reps
Lunge with a Twist (both sides)	15 reps each side

Day 17

Warm Up Exercise: Mindful Breathing

Somatic Exercises	Reps
Plank	35 seconds
Bridge Pose	25 seconds
Jumping Jacks	4 minutes
Balancing Table Pose (both sides)	15 reps each side
Lunge with a Twist (both	12 reps each side

sides)	
Shoulder Circles	25 reps

Day 18

Warm Up Exercise: Gentle Head Rolls

Somatic Exercises	Reps
Wall Push-Ups	30 reps
Knee-to-Chest Stretches (both sides)	20 reps each side
Arm Circles	30 reps
Jogging on the Spot	6 minutes
Side Plank Variations (both sides)	45 seconds each side

Day 19

Warm Up Exercise: Shoulder Circles

Somatic Exercises	**Reps**
Glute and Hip Flexor Activation (both sides)	20 reps each side
Breath Awareness Exercise	7 minutes
Calf Muscle Stretching (both sides)	25 seconds each side
Single-Leg Deadlift with Overhead Reach (both sides)	18 reps each side
Ankle Stability Exercises	20 reps
Core Rotations (both sides)	20 reps each side

Day 20

Warm Up Exercise: Spinal Twists

Somatic Exercises	**Reps**

Pilates-Inspired Ab Workouts	20 reps
Squats	30 reps
Lunge with a Twist (both sides)	18 reps each side
Plank	40 seconds
Bridge Pose	30 seconds
Jumping Jacks	5 minutes

Day 21

Warm Up Exercise: Mindful Breathing

Somatic Exercises	Reps
Balancing Table Pose (both sides)	18 reps each side

Lunge with a Twist (both sides)	15 reps each side
Shoulder Circle	30 reps
Wall Push-Ups	35 reps
Knee-to-Chest Stretches (both sides)	25 reps each side
Arm Circles	35 reps

Week 4

Day 22

Warm Up Exercise: Spinal Twists

Somatic Exercises	Reps
Jogging on the Spot	8 minutes
Side Plank Variations (both sides)	55 seconds each side

Glute and Hip Flexor Activation (both sides)	25 reps each side
Breath Awareness Exercise	8 minutes
Calf Muscle Stretching (both sides)	30 seconds each side

Day 23

Warm Up Exercise: Mindful Breathing

Somatic Exercises	Reps
Single-Leg Deadlift with Overhead Reach (both sides)	20 reps each side
Ankle Stability Exercises	25 reps
Core Rotations (both sides)	25 reps each side
Pilates-Inspired Ab Workouts	25 reps

Squats	35 reps
Lunge with a Twist (both sides)	20 reps each side

Day 24

Warm Up Exercise: Gentle Head Rolls

Somatic Exercises	Reps
Bridge Pose	35 seconds
Jumping Jacks	6 minutes
Balancing Table Pose (both sides)	20 reps each side
Lunge with a Twist (both sides)	18 reps each side
Shoulder Circles	35 reps
Wall Push-Ups	40 reps

Day 25

Warm Up Exercise: Shoulder Circles

Somatic Exercises	Reps
Knee-to-Chest Stretches (both sides)	30 reps each side
Arm Circles	40 reps
Jogging on the Spot	10 minutes
Plank	45 seconds
Side Plank Variations (both sides)	60 seconds each side

Day 26

Warm Up Exercise: Spinal Twists

Somatic Exercises	Reps

Glute and Hip Flexor Activation (both sides)	30 reps each side
Breath Awareness Exercise	10 minutes
Calf Muscle Stretching (both sides)	35 seconds each side
Single-Leg Deadlift with Overhead Reach (both sides)	25 reps each side
Ankle Stability Exercises	30 reps
Core Rotations (both sides)	30 reps each side

Day 27

Warm Up Exercise: Mindful Breathing

Somatic Exercises	Reps
Pilates-Inspired Ab Workouts	30 reps

Squats	40 reps
Lunge with a Twist (both sides)	25 reps each side
Plank	50 seconds
Bridge Pose	40 seconds
Jumping Jacks	8 minutes

Day 28

Warm Up Exercise: Gentle Head Rolls

Somatic Exercises	Reps
Balancing Table Pose (both sides)	25 reps each side
Lunge with a Twist (both sides)	20 reps each side
Shoulder Circles	40 reps

Wall Push-Ups	45 reps
Knee-to-Chest Stretches (both sides)	35 reps each side
Arm Circles	45 reps

CONCLUSION

As we come to the conclusion of "Somatic Exercises for Weight Loss," let's take a moment to look back at the journey we've shared. This book has been more than a guide for losing weight; it's been a holistic exploration of well-being, blending physical, mental, and nutritional aspects of health. From the beginning, we dived into the world of somatic exercises, where mindful movement and body awareness come together. These exercises go beyond just physical fitness; they're about creating a deeper understanding and connection with your body.-

Throughout this book, themes of persistence and adaptability have echoed. The path to well-being isn't always straightforward; it's a journey marked with challenges and victories. The routines and advice provided give you a framework but are flexible to adjust to your evolving needs and circumstances. In this journey, every small step matters, and each bit of progress is worth celebrating. -

As you continue on your wellness path, remember that it's a journey of self-discovery and enhancement. Your relationship with your body is personal, requiring patience, dedication, and compassion. The road to well-being is ongoing, and along the way, you'll discover more about yourself, your strengths, and areas for growth. Embrace the spirit of this journey by maintaining the practices and principles you've learned here. Keep exploring somatic exercises, listen to your body's cues, nourish it thoughtfully, and, above all, approach your well-being journey with kindness and an open heart.- - -

www.ingramcontent.com/pod-product-compliance
Lightning Source LLC
Chambersburg PA
CBHW070819280726
48660CB00016B/2140